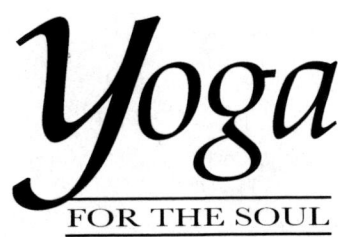

Yoga
FOR THE SOUL

The Wisdom of Yoga for Everyday Life

Learn more about the author at www.BecomingPeace.Net
Design, photography and illustration by Cynthia Koelsch Design Inc.
Author's Photo: Richard Ehrlick
National Library of Canada Cataloguing in Publication
Arbic, Neal.
Yoga for the Soul: The Wisdom of Yoga for Everyday Life / Neal Arbic
Little Lotus Press

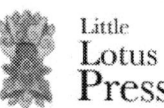

© Copyright 2005 Neal Arbic.

All rights reserved. No part of this publication may be reproduced, stored in a retrieval system, or transmitted, in any form or by any means, electronic, mechanical, photocopying, recording, or otherwise, without the written prior permission of the author.

Note for Librarians: A cataloguing record for this book is available from Library and Archives Canada at www.collectionscanada.ca/amicus/index-e.html
ISBN 1-4120-3902-9

Printed in Victoria, BC, Canada. Printed on paper with minimum 30% recycled fibre. Trafford's print shop runs on "green energy" from solar, wind and other environmentally-friendly power sources.

TRAFFORD

Offices in Canada, USA, Ireland and UK

Trafford Publishing, 6E–2333 Government St.,
Victoria, BC v8t 4p4 CANADA
phone 250 383 6864 (toll-free 1 888 232 4444)
fax 250 383 6804; email to orders@trafford.com

Trafford Publishing (UK) Ltd., Enterprise House, Wistaston Road Business Centre,
Wistaston Road, Crewe, Cheshire cw2 7rp UNITED KINGDOM
phone 01270 251 396 (local rate 0845 230 9601)
facsimile 01270 254 983; orders.uk@trafford.com
Order online at:
trafford.com/04-1710

10 9 8 7 6 5 4 3

This book is dedicated to

Ram Dass
who showed me the path
&
Babaji
(Baba Hari Dass)
who showed me how to walk it.

Introduction

When I was 23 I had it all: a record contract, a movie deal, fans and groupies. I was a star. And I was absolutely miserable.

Before I would think, "I'll be happy when... I get a contract, a movie deal...", but what happens when you have got it all and you're still unhappy?

In the end, I left it all behind. For two years I looked for answers in every religion and holy person I could find, but no one seemed real.
Then, almost by accident, I met an Indian monk. His very being changed my life. Baba Hari Dass had a radiant inner peace I could feel. For the next sixteen years, he taught me the philosophy of yoga.

These ideas were presented to me as "ideas". I was not asked to join a group, or give money. So now I offer them in this spirit. If you find these ideas useful, please take them. If they seem wrong, by all means, reject them. Consider this book a buffet; take only what you like.

I share these words because they have brought me great peace, again and again.

So find a quiet space, make a cup of tea and sit with these words. Pause every now and then. Let them enter your heart, and fill your soul.

Peace,

Neal

*"Better than a thousand words,
is a few words that bring peace"*
- The Buddha

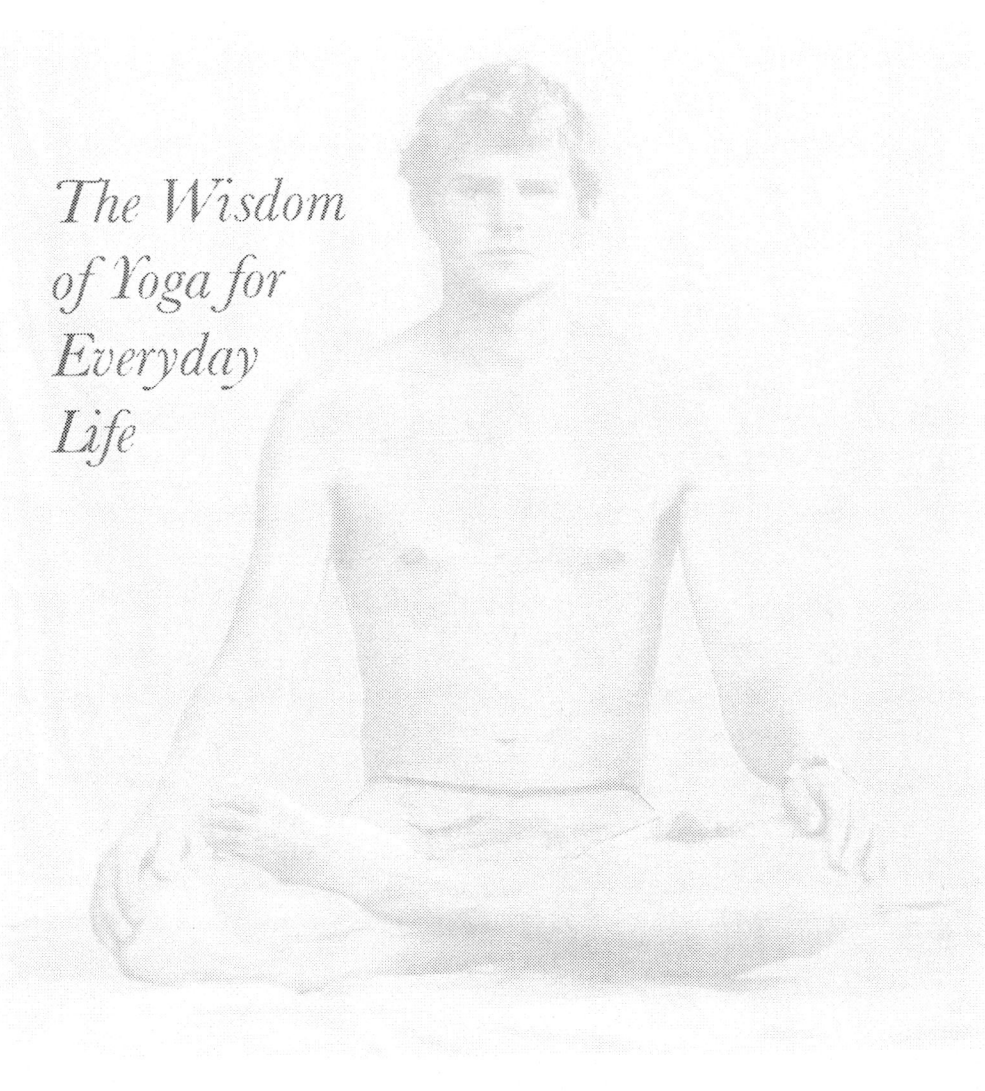

The Wisdom of Yoga for Everyday Life

We create our own reality.

*Our thoughts,
words and actions
create our destinies.
It is our inner attitudes
that shape our outer experiences.*

Love
   Peace
      Compassion

*When our thoughts and actions
   come from these feelings,*

   the world answers us with:

   Love
      Peace
         Compassion

Our inner attitudes create the world we live in.

Have you ever acted with a selfish, uncaring attitude?

*People didn't go
"Wow, we love YOU!"
The attitude came right back at you.*

We reap what we sow.

And we can't fake it.

Like...

I'm acting nice because I want you to be nice to me.

That's not real nice.

*People know
when it comes from your heart
and when you're expecting
something
in return.*

*On some level they can tell
if you're playing a game,*

even if you don't.

Karma Karma Karma

We are the world.
   It's that simple.

        If your heart is full of desires
        how can you be
        happy?

                You'll see a world
                full of limitations
                and obstacles.

*When your heart is free of all desire
how can you not be happy?*

*You'll see a world
just as it is:
limitless
and free.*

PERFECT
*the way
it is.*

As we feel,
                so we see.

How we see,
                is how we act.

How we act,
                creates the response;

      that response

  is the world we live in.

The moment you give it up...

everything

falls

into

place.

A good heart sows peace.
A bad heart brings trouble.

That's it.

Have you ever been here?

I'LL BE HAPPY WHEN...

I GET WHAT I WANT,

HOW I WANT IT,

WHEN I WANT IT.

                    UNTIL THEN, I HAVE THE RIGHT
                            TO BE AS MISERABLE
                                  AS I WANT.

The more you want...
the less likely you are to be happy.

The less you want....
the more happy you're likely to be.

Here we go...

*I once asked Babaji
why I didn't feel
God was always with me.*

He said,

"Your mind is too outwardly".

You know the game:

THE ANSWER IS OUT THERE SOMEWHERE

> Happiness is...
> - a new car,
> - a bigger house,
> - a new job.
>
> Whatever I don't have **NOW**.
> Always the bigger, better deal.
>
> Always looking for some thing:
> I can do, own, achieve.

*You can look for abiding happiness
outside of yourself.*

*But sooner or later
you find
out:*

It doesn't last.

Because:

Nothing lasts.

*There's no permanent ground
outside of your soul.*

*In the material realm
the only permanent thing is...*

Change

You get old;
Things burn down;
People leave or die.

Because it's all…

Impermanent

One day you're on top

and then you're not.

That's it.

THAT'S THE WORLD.

You can chain all your hopes and dreams on that,
however
be prepared to be tossed

back & forth,

up
&
down.

This feels great! *This is really painful.*
I won! *I lost.*
I'm great! *I suck.*
Everyone is loving me! *No one cares about me.*
Good news! *Bad news.*
Good news! *Bad news.*
Really Good news! *Really Bad news.*

It never ends...

Because:

**It's all castles made of sand,
falling into the sea.**

So...

*Where is the answer?
Where is peace?
Lasting happiness?*

All the Prophets,

all the Gurus,

all the Buddha's,

Messiahs and Saints,

they all say the same thing:

Look within.

Deep inside
there's a quiet space within you,

and it just watches,
watches everything:

the world,
us.

It's you!

not your body,

not your mind,

your soul.

Everything you've been looking for;

it's right there.

*And that 'you' isn't Joe Smith
who lives at 144 Moonbeam St.
who likes ice cream and baseball.*

That's your mind!

*Your soul is...
well...*

It's... beyond, beyond...

You have to go there to find out

**because it's beyond thoughts,
beyond words.**

*No one else can tell you
because words and ideas have limits
and...*

the soul is...

limitless

So you have to take the journey.

You know...

THE WAY, THE PATH
Your soul's been waiting all along.

Quietly waiting for you...

for:

when the mind is quiet
the soul is revealed.

If you sat and meditated everyday for ten years
If you prayed throughout the stillness of the night
If you started to take a little quiet time just

      to reflect

      to fast

      to look inwards

      you would see who you really are.

            You would find...

Nirvana

God

No matter what you call it...

The Tao

The Self

The Oneness of the Soul

That's who you are.

*Under all your fears and desires,
under all your stuff
(and it's just stuff)*

That's who you are.

Different words?
 Same idea.

   Different ideas?
      Same experience.

Have you ever...
screwed up?
And yet deep down inside you knew it all the time.

That quiet space inside
was telling you
"You're doing something wrong.
You're headed away from happiness."

But you ignored it.

Because of
　　desire
　　　or ego
　　　　or something you were attached to
　　　　　you said:

"Other people do it. So who cares."

But deep down inside...

　　you started to feel
　　　　unhappy;
　　　　　uneasy?

Mind thinks.

Soul knows.

*And that's the difference between
being pleasantly distracted
&
finding happiness.*

So we begin that journey to inner peace;

*to that peace which was there
before our bodies were
formed*
&
*that will be there long
after our bodies have
dissolved.*

*And to experience it… now.
On steady ground…*

The Sanctuary of the Soul.

Many people have faith.
    Many people believe.
        They start the journey,
            but then they get
                lost along the way.

They memorize Scripture,
and then just argue to show off their knowledge.

    People do yoga,
    and turn it into a competition.

*People pray or meditate
and think they're better than those who don't.*

*People get totally devoted to their faiths
and hate (even kill) others who see God differently.*

*Many are called,
but few go all the way.*

after all...

It's tempting, to translate

God into our world.

To make Love and Peace

into some thing:

we can own,

belong to,

or possess.

We want another object

to make us feel better.

Because... it's so much harder to....

really

change

and...

Surrender
   to God

*So we end up changing God. But these games don't
work, sooner or later the house of cards
collapses. Because we build it on
our egos, our desires and
attachments. And
ultimately, this
is what made
us unhappy
in the first
place.*

Here's the deal

DESIRE
is a part of life.

*But on the other hand,
when it's not fulfilled, it's awful:
the disappointment, frustration and anger.*

Desire becomes a trap...

It creates a gulf between

Us

&

Happiness

I'LL BE HAPPY *WHEN*...
• I WIN A MILLION BUCKS
• I GET HOME
• YOU CLEAN YOUR ROOM

Dissatisfaction
is the shadow of desire.

*One
can't arise without
the other.*

It's a mixed bag.

ATTACHMENT
also seems great.

You love your family, house, car.
It's great, until you lose them.

Then it's painful.

*The mere thought of it
creates worry and fear.*

*That awful anxiety.
That terrible pain of loss.*

*You wish it could last forever,
but it doesn't.*

*And the deeper you are attached,
the deeper you grieve.*

Another mixed bag.

EGO
so worshipped by so many,

and it's wonderful to feel accomplished.
And yet, all the times when people put you down,
the pain of shame, insults, jealousy,
that's all part of the deal too.

The concept of 'me' and 'mine'
is behind all the conflicts that
tear our world apart.

*All the sufferings
of desire and attachment
are all expressions of
ego:
that sense of separation
from others
&
everything.*

*As hard as we try,
(and it's all we really do)
we can't separate pain from pleasure.*

It's two sides of the same coin of Ego.

*On one side there's life
and on the other there's death.*

*It's a packaged deal:
Life & Death*

*That's the realm we're so attached to.
It's where we build our homes,
hopes and dreams.*

Does it seem like a wise investment?

*No matter how much you get,
one day you're going to lose it all;*

even your body,

even your mind.

Then what?

Do we know who we are?
Have we taken that journey?
Do we know what nothingness is like?

Or

Are we too busy trying to win the game
no one can win?

*You don't have to give it all up
and live in a cave.*

You need only realize:

We create our own suffering

*through
ego, desire
and attachment.*

So...

Give these up.

*Look at what you have to do
in the world
as simply
your duty.*

Do your duty,

but give the results up to The Divine.

Do your work!
And forget about the rewards.

Do the right thing
*   for your family,*
*   community.*

But give up your
*   worry, hate,*
*   frustrations,*
*   and expectations.*

Act on love

Live in faith

after all...

It's just a drama
the mind is caught up in.

*But if you're watching it all,
even yourself, from that
quiet inner space
in the eternal*

*then you see
there's no big deal,
Nothing really matters.
Nothing is really happening.*

And that
'detachment'

that lack of
'selfishness'

*allows you
under all circumstances,
to do the right thing.*

And not be:

deluded by your
EGO

swayed by your
DESIRES

or blinded by your
ATTACHMENTS

But to do what's best for everyone.

You act on

God's behalf.

That is Love...
and all its many faces:

Peace

Truth

Justice

Clarity

Charity

Sacrifice

Compassion

Non-violent resistance

To live love
&
not be led astray.

*But how do we connect to Love
when we're out
in the world
and on
the go?*

We come back home

*to where we are
&
what we're doing.*

To see it again, as if for the first time.

Seeing through the
EGO

Getting past
DESIRES

and without
ATTACHMENT

Just doing what needs to be done

Here and now.

No thought of future reward.

Peace is not in the future:
The future is just your imagination.
You can't show it to me.
Where is it?

Peace is not the past.
The past is just memory,
Only the relics and pictures remain.
How can we find peace in what doesn't even exist?

If you are looking for peace....

IT'S HERE RIGHT NOW

We've always been "Here".
No matter where you are,
you'll always be Here.

Eternity is "Now".
It's always been Now
and it will always
be Now.

It's right in front of our eyes.

It's been there all along.

That's not the world you're looking at.

It's God:

The Eternal Now;

The Limitless Here.

So...

*Don't worry,
be happy.*

Take care
of the present moment.
That's all you have to do.
No big drama.

But...

if you can't...see that

everyone
&
everything

is God.

Then there's still more yoga to do.

*It's always a matter of purity.
You can't get away from it.*

It takes a pure heart to see God.

*It takes a lot of virtue
to find abiding happiness.*

PEACE
from Virtue;

VIRTUE
from Discipline.

Now,
most everyone wants peace.

most everyone respects virtue.
(Even criminals in prison rank themselves
according to their crimes.)

It's
Discipline
that's the bummer.

It's hard to deal peacefully with those who irritate you.
It's hard to make time for meditation every day.
It's not always easy to 'be here now'

it can be hard to remember.

*And sometimes being good
doesn't always pay off
in worldly ways.*

*You
"do good"*

&

someone gets upset.

Make no mistake about it.

It's a challenge,

getting

free.

As long as we are on the level of ego,

there will be suffering!

But your choice is to make it...

MEANINGFUL or MEANINGLESS?

Meaningless suffering (meéninglis súfəring)

n. **1.** harming yourself and others and denying it or never learning from the experience. **2.** unnecessary suffering leading to more useless suffering with no end in sight. **3.** getting what you want, losing what you want; making enemies along the way.

On the other hand,

Meaningful suffering (meéningfool súfəring)

n. **1.** the challenge of discipline has an aim; a purpose. **2.** to be good; **3.** to be as holy as you can muster at the moment; so as to...

PURIFY

all within you that makes you suffer.

And by doing so reaching

The end of suffering.

*Like
Jesus on
the
cross.
He's not swearing at what
a bad day he's having. He's surrendering
to God! He's merging into God. There's no ego
saying "I want to live. How can you do this to ME!"*

Because...

He's pure; He's giving up

the individual Ego

for

the universal One.

No DESIRE or ATTACHMENT

And all that's left is ...

Love

*He's asking God
to forgive those who are killing him:*

The End Of Suffering

No ego = No suffering

You don't have to suffer.

You don't have to live with problems.

You can always choose option C:

    a) Get revenge

    b) Give up

c) Be Happy Now

because if you wait...

    you'll wait forever.

If...

*you meditated every day
for one year.*

*You'd begin to find
that peaceful space within you.*

*That place where all this worldly stuff
cannot reach.*

*You'd begin to feel that quiet energy entering
into your day.*

*That peace becomes a perfect reference point;
A refuge from the storm.*

*Sometimes,
your meditations will show you
things you'd rather not see,*

like your selfishness.

*But you deal with that in meditation
instead of dragging it out into the day
so everyone can suffer.*

As you begin to purify,
your heart becomes lighter, your mind clearer.

And as the burdens of ego, desires and attachment
start to thin,

you start to feel more connected,
to that loving, peaceful space.

But watch out!

Ego always finds a way to cash in on virtue. You've got to watch that ego! If you start "doing good", watch it doesn't become:

"I" did good.

*Then it stops being a
'giving up of everything to God'*

and becomes

"Look at me I'm so holy!"

*"How dare you treat me that way!
Can't you see I'm holy ?!"*

It's a tricky game.

"Do you go all the way?"

Or do you settle for what's behind door number two?

Life is not always fair,

        but it's going to happen anyway.

The question is,

"How much are you going to suffer?"

      In the end,

          it's up to you.

                After all,

We create our own reality.

I have failed miserably so many times at being a yogi and I'm still not one yet. But, I've never given up. And that's the way it works. You won't be Mother Teresa by next Friday, the latest. So enjoy the struggle.

Because sometimes, it's a struggle.

But it has its rewards. There is a real joy in freedom: in not getting caught in the world; not being trapped by desire; catching yourself getting lost and being able to return to the present moment.

Finding yourself helping, instead of hurting.

Telling the truth.
Keeping the peace.

Giving up a desire for the sake of just being a better person.

A little self-mastery...   can go a long way.

And then suddenly

*You're happy
deep, deep down inside.*

It's not like you found happiness.
You are happiness.

It's not like someone gave you peace.
You are peace.

*And no matter how many times you fail,
you can always come back.*

For ours is not a journey of sorrow.

So rejoice!

No matter how many times you have fallen,

"REJOICE!"

And come...   *come again.*

Leave

sorrow

behind.

The past is gone
&
the future will never arrive.

So practice peace... now.

The best you can

and you will see...

*the moment
you don't want a thing*

is the moment...

you have it all

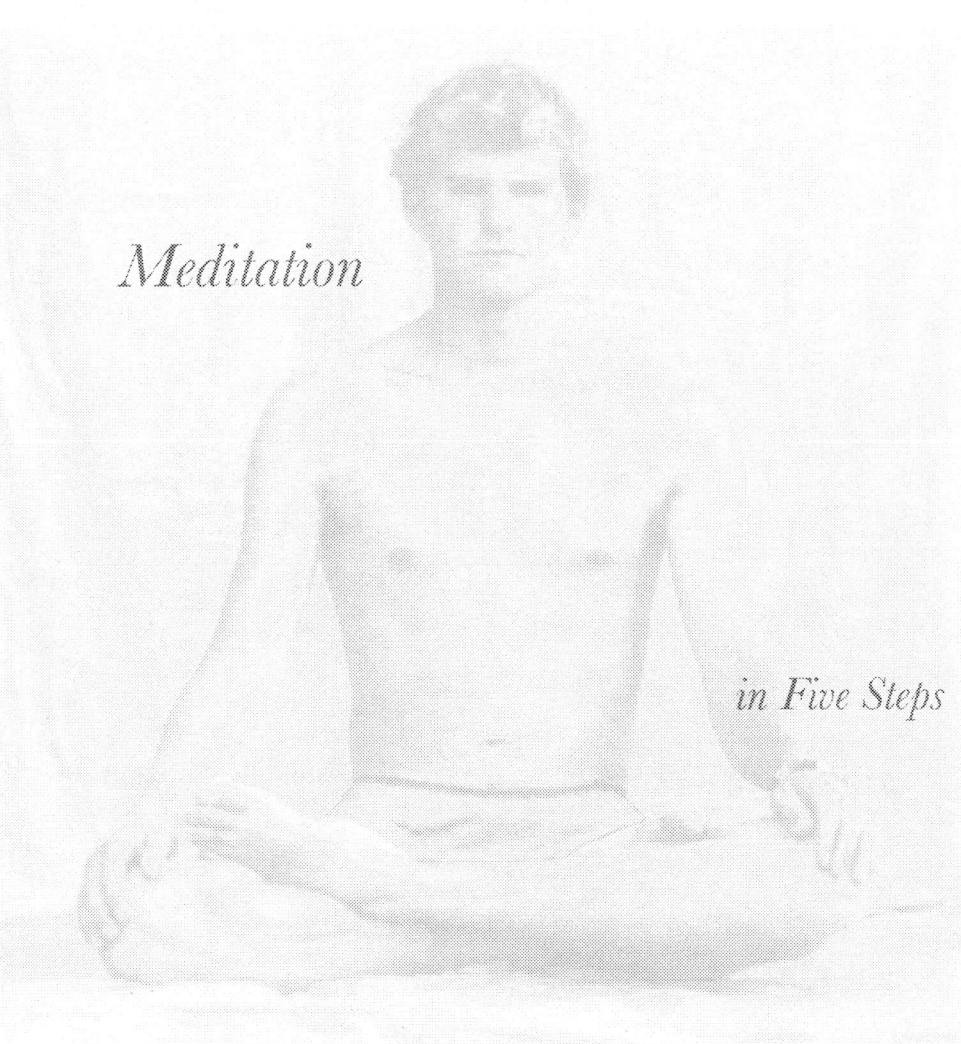

Find a comfortable Posture

*Your head, neck and spine should be in a
straight line without feeling rigid.
Let the spine relax upwards.
Loosen your clothing if possible.
The tongue rests lightly on the roof of the mouth.
Sitting cross-legged on a blanket or a pillow is
traditional and calming, but standing, lying down
or sitting in a chair is fine.*

NOTE: *If you sit on the floor, place a rolled blanket or cushion behind you
slightly under the tailbone, so you can sit with the spine staight.*

Relax the abdomen

When you really let go of the belly,
you can feel the breath moving within it.
Then the rest of the body will automatically relax.
Allow the belly, "the seat of tension"
within your body, to become your
"centre of relaxation".

Gently focus the mind on the breath

This is not a hard concentration that will give you a headache. Have a relaxed awareness of every inhalation and exhalation. Let the mind "watch" the breath, not control it. Allow the mind to "rest" in this awareness of breath.

NOTE: If the breath leaves the abdomen and becomes shallow, that is fine as long as the breath is calm, slow and gentle (quiet). Simply rest the mind in the sensation of breathing.

*When the mind wanders from the breath
gently bring it back*

*The mind will not always want to stay in this
peaceful awareness.
It will want to do more exciting things
like worry or daydream.
When it does... smile, relax and bring it back.*

Relax and enjoy

*Meditation should be a release, a letting go
of pressure and worry, not a judgement
on how many times your mind wandered away.
Let it go... let it be.
Don't push thoughts away or cling to them.
Just let them float by like clouds in the sky.
Ignore them, as you take the time to enjoy
the beautiful feeling... of simply breathing.*

Meditation Opportunities:

Traffic jams, line ups, subway rides,
waiting for a bus, plane, doctor, etc.

Tense situations:
Release the abdomen, become aware of your breath.

Meditating daily gets the best results,
but even a little practice can bring good results.
Early morning or evening is traditional.
Start with 10 minutes, then 20.
With time you will naturally want to stay longer.

*NOTE: Every couple of days meditate without the CD.
If your surroundings are noisy, you can use ear plugs.*

There are many other objects suitable for meditation

*A traditional Yogic meditation is to visualize
the full moon at Anja Charka,
the third eye between the eye brows.*

*The visualization of the soul,
seen as a flame glowing within the centre of the chest,
the heart chakra, is yet another form of meditation.*

*Mantra: a repeated phrase
or sound. The famous
"aum" can be repeated
mentally.*

The Ideal

The ideal is to hold the object one-pointedly,
just like you would hold a new born baby.
One holds a baby with great care and attention,
but also with an attitude of loving affection.
One should embrace and merge with the object.

Sit still,
do nothing.
Don't try to get enlightened, don't try to get inner peace -
no "getting."
Just sit. Let the mind rest in the object.
You are peace. Just let the dust of the mind settle and you will feel it.

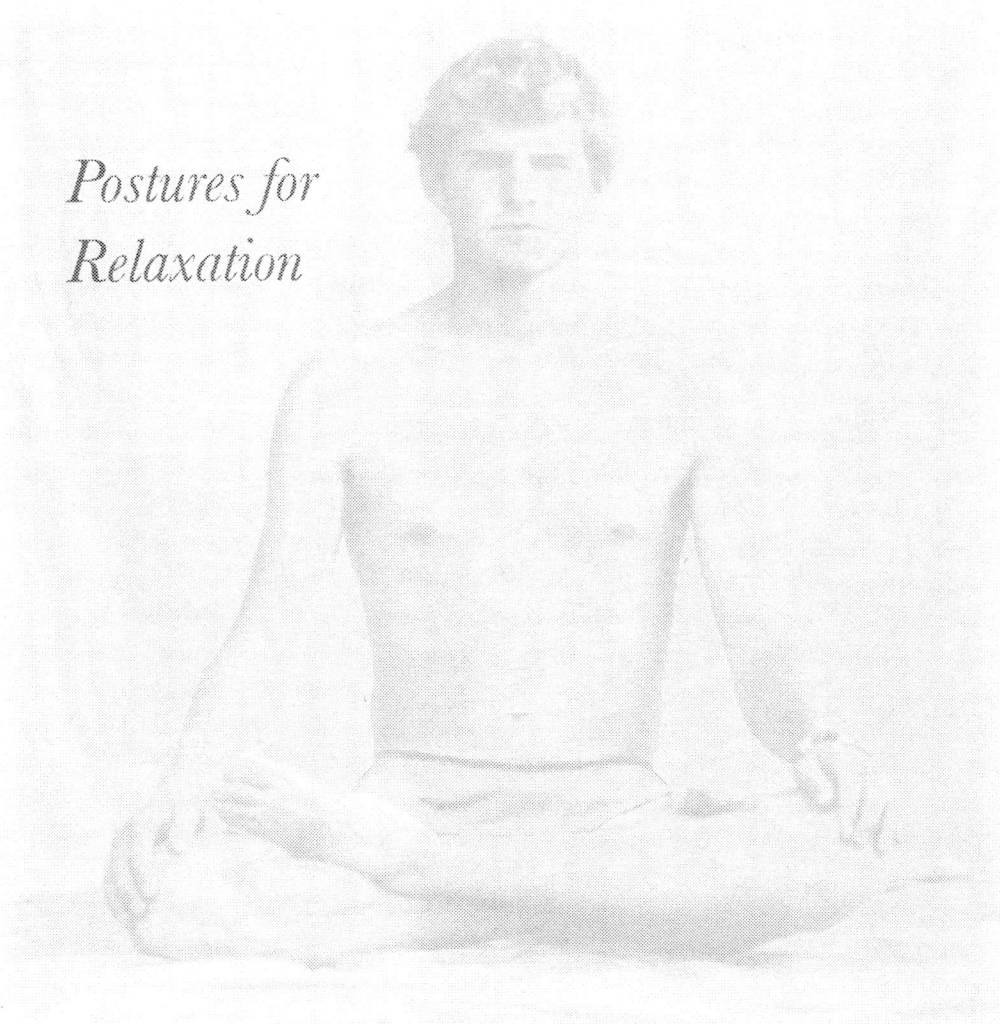

Postures for Relaxation

This is a relaxing form of yoga that everyone should be able to do. The poses are shown for beginners, but if you know the more advanced forms, feel free to practice them. Once you are familiar with the poses, you do not have to follow the CD step by step; you can go right into the poses and hold them longer as you would in an advanced class.

Consult your physician before beginning this or any exercise program, especially if you have any of the following conditions:

Neck pain
Lower back problems
Disc problems
Pregnancy
High blood pressure
Hiatus hernia
Glaucoma
Heart problems
Stroke

Preparation:

*Find a warm, well-ventilated room
where you can relax undisturbed.*

Wear loose comfortable clothing.

Put a mat or a folded blanket on the floor.

*Have an empty stomach for practice.
A drink just before practice is fine.
Wait 2 to 3 hours after a meal.*

Take a restroom break before you begin.

Introduction

How do we do the poses?
If I had to sum it up in one word it would be "relaxed".

The aim of Yoga is peace. The Yoga Sutras say,
"The perfection of posture is the relaxation of tension",
or
in Yoga the perfect stretch is the relaxed one.

Over stretching and feeling pain is dangerous.
Under-stretching and feeling nothing achieves few benefits.
So, how do you know when your stretch is just right?
When it feels good.

It's not like a gymnastics stretch where it's all
about looking good on the outside. It's about how it feels, to you,
on the inside. The stretch should be pleasant and steady.

*In Yoga, we work with the body, not against it.
Poses can "hurt-so-good" -a pleasant discomfort.
But if you're in pain and you can't relax the stretch, you've gone too far.*

*Yoga is an exercise for the body and mind.
You should always, in every pose, be aware of how you feel.
The mind gently concentrates on the feeling and the breath.
In this way our practice becomes a meditation:
calming and strengthening the body and mind.*

To sum it up in three rules:

*1. Go in and out of the postures slowly.
2. Stretch only so far as feels good (or at least not painful)
3. Come out of the pose when it starts to feel uncomfortable.
Tune in to how you feel; No pain, no strain.*

The Yoga Poses

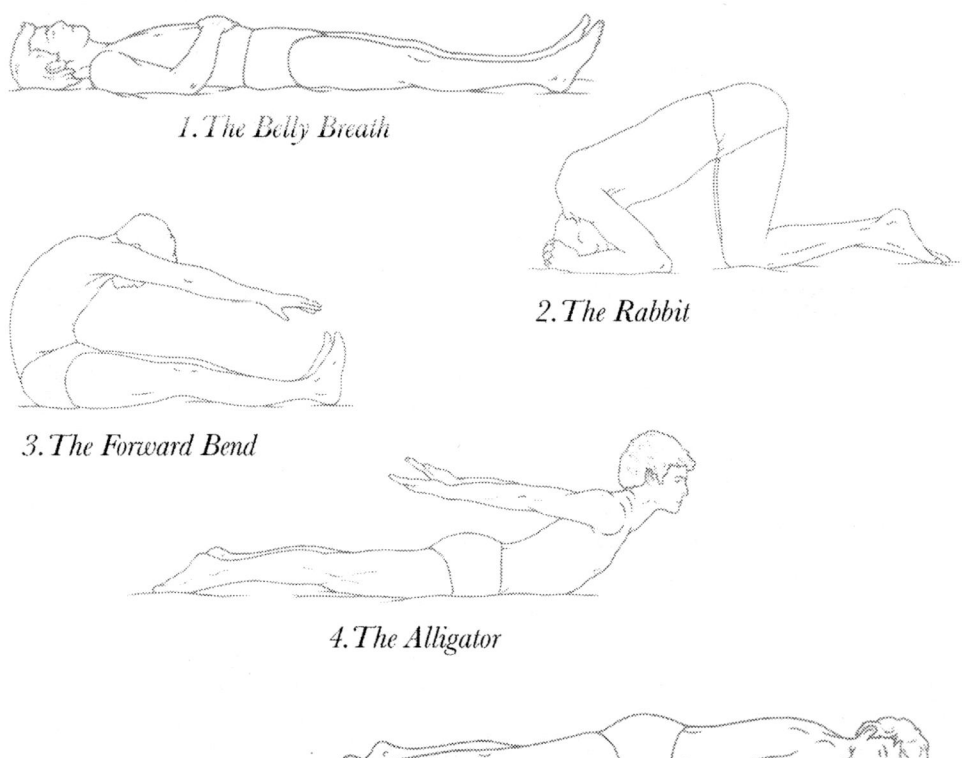

1. The Belly Breath
2. The Rabbit
3. The Forward Bend
4. The Alligator
5. The Reverse Relaxation

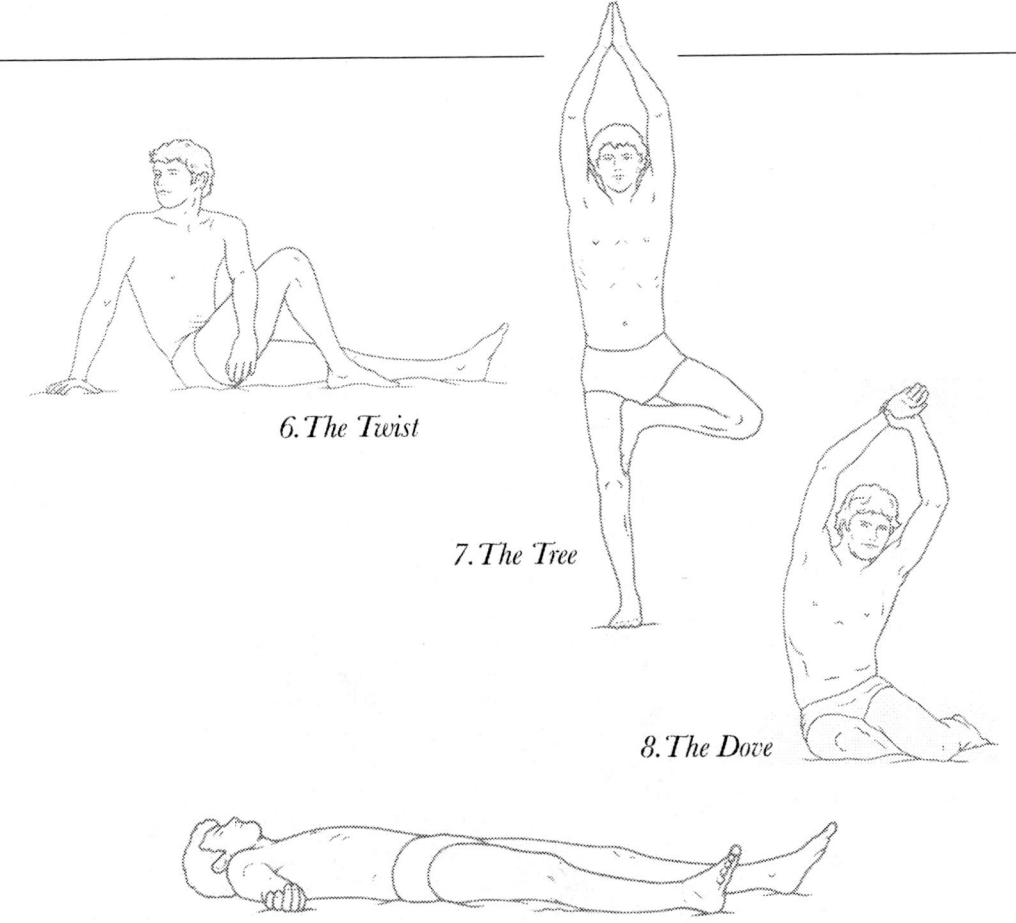

6. The Twist

7. The Tree

8. The Dove

9. The Final Relaxation

The Belly Breath

The Pose

Lie on the back. Let the feet fall apart so legs are relaxed.
Legs just far enough apart so the lower back is free of pressure.
To release the arms and neck, lift the shoulders slightly, put them down
slowly. Relax the jaw where it meets the ears. Drop the tongue to the back
of the mouth. Let the eyes become soft, unfocused, like in sleep. Place one
hand on the abdomen,
just above the
belly button
- just below
the rib cage.

Relax the
abdomen
so the breath
is free and easy.

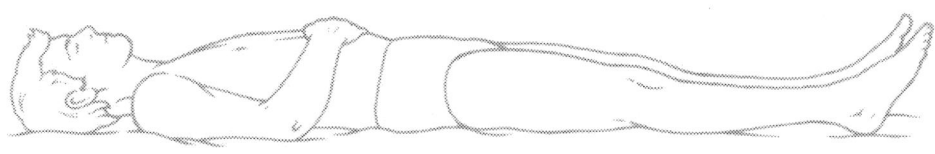

The Feel

If the abdomen is soft, you will feel the hand rising with the inhale and falling with the exhale. Do not control this movement. Release the abdomen and it will happen naturally. Let the mind rest in this feeling - the gentle movement of the breath, like waves washing upon a beach, and back out again.

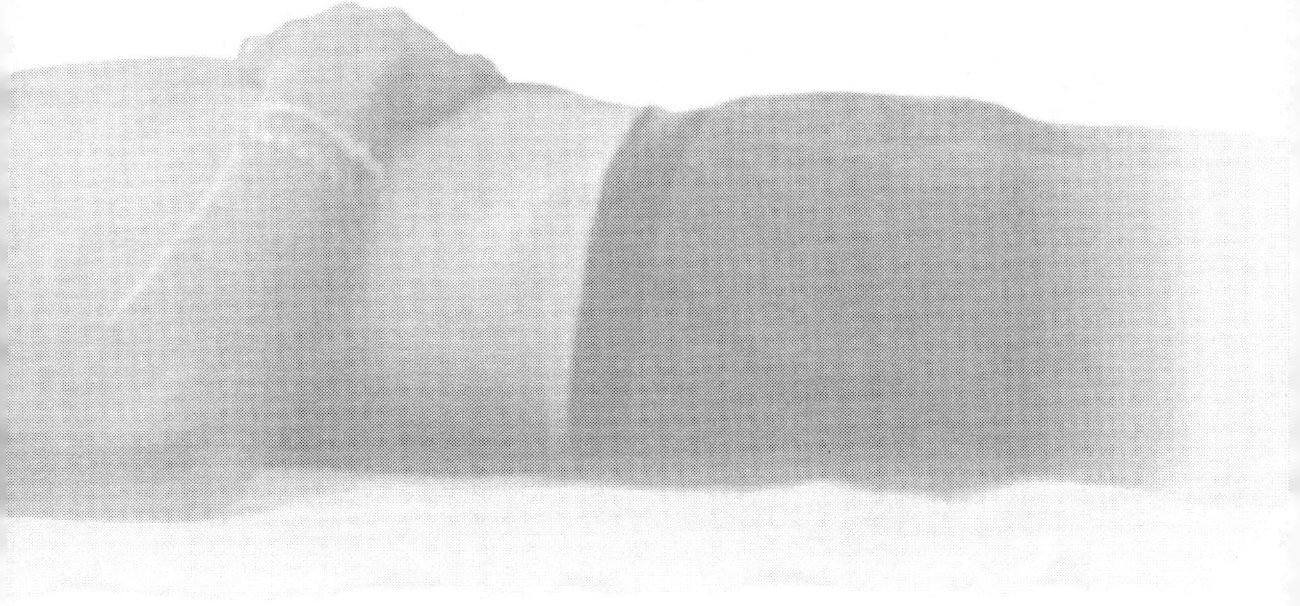

The Rabbit

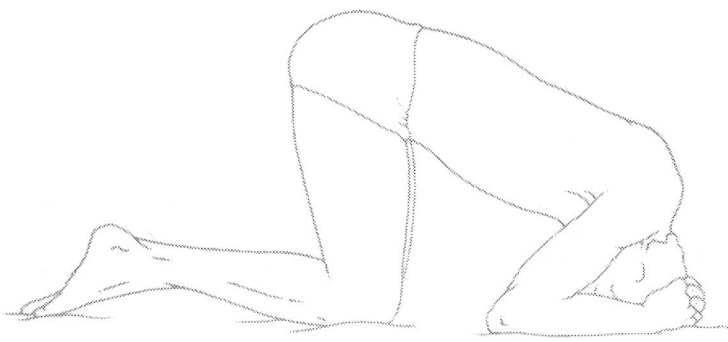

The Pose
Come onto the knees and elbows
(elbows underneath the shoulders, knees under the hips).
Interlock the fingers. Place the top of the head on the
floor in front of the hands. (You should feel the
hands touching the back of your head.)

Tip: *If you have high blood pressure,
glaucoma or neck problems you can
rest the forehead on top of the hands.*

The Feel

Use the arms to control the pressure on the head and especially the neck. Release the abdomen and let the body sink into the pose.

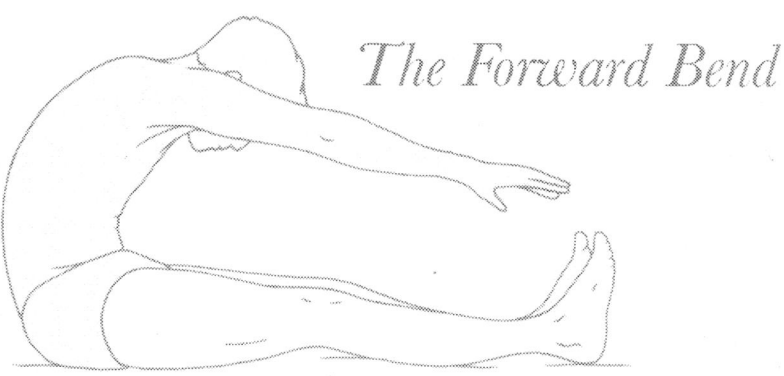

The Forward Bend

The Pose

Sit with the legs together out in front of you. Like a yawn, stretch the arms up over the head. With an exhalation, while keeping the back straight, fold the hips forward over the legs.

Stage one:

When the hips stop, round the back. Don't reach out yet. Let the hands drop where they naturally fall on the legs. Relax, as soft as a rag doll. Let the shoulder blades fall apart. Take a moment to let the body open.

Stage two:

With an exhalation, point the toes back towards the head and reach out towards the feet. Hands are high in the air, above toe level. Look down at the knees, not up at how far you are stretching.

Hold as long as feels good. With an inhalation, come up.

The Feel

Fold forward from the hips, (you should feel the sitting bones in the buttocks move back, the pelvis tilts down towards the floor.) The idea is not to touch your toes, but to gently stretch the back of body from the legs up to the neck.

When reaching out, keep the shoulders wide, so you don't crunch the neck.

The Alligator

The Pose

Come onto the stomach,
legs together, arms at the side, palms turned up.
Squeeze the buttocks together and push the hips down.

With an inhalation,
lift the chest and arms.
Hold for a moment.
With an exhalation,
release down.

Tip: *Keep the buttocks tight throughout the pose; this protects the lower back.*

The Feel

The spine gently stretches out and away from the hip.

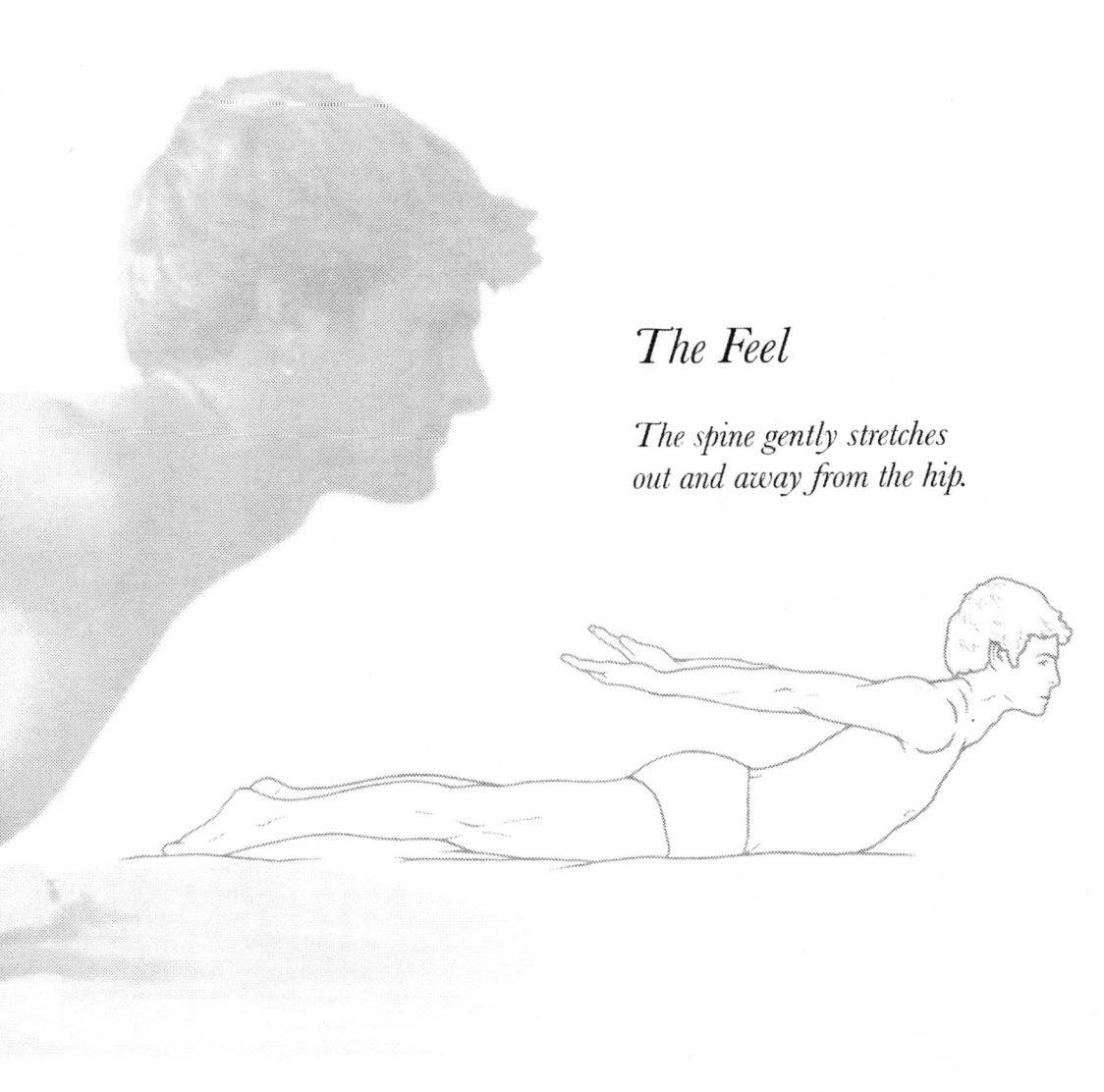

The Reverse Relaxation

The Pose

*Lie on the belly.
Turn you head to one side,
resting on a cheek bone.*

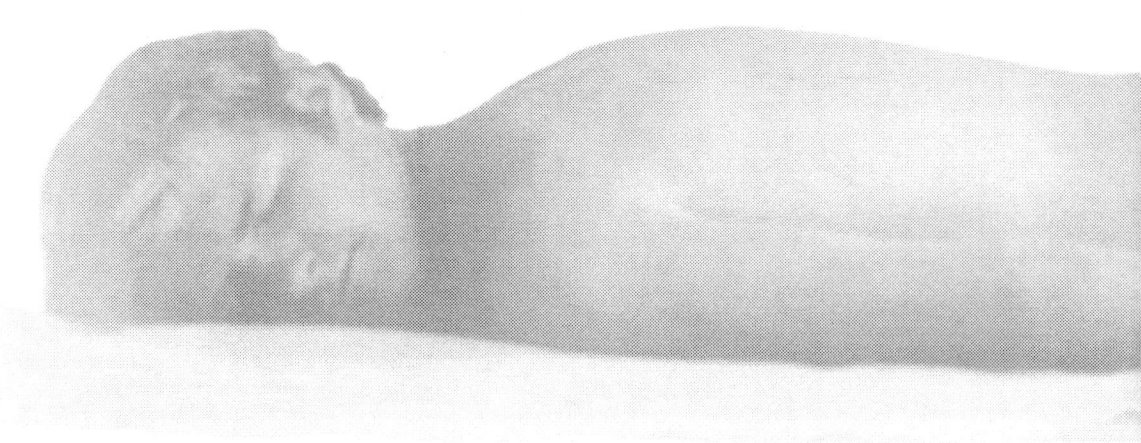

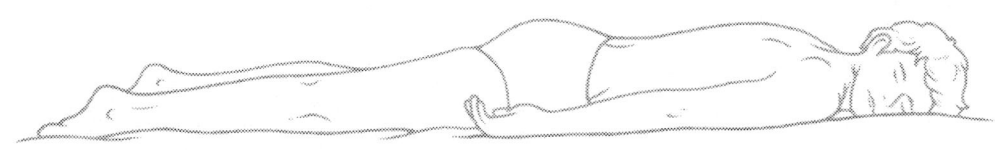

The Feel

Relax the upper back, the neck and even the face, as if you are falling asleep.

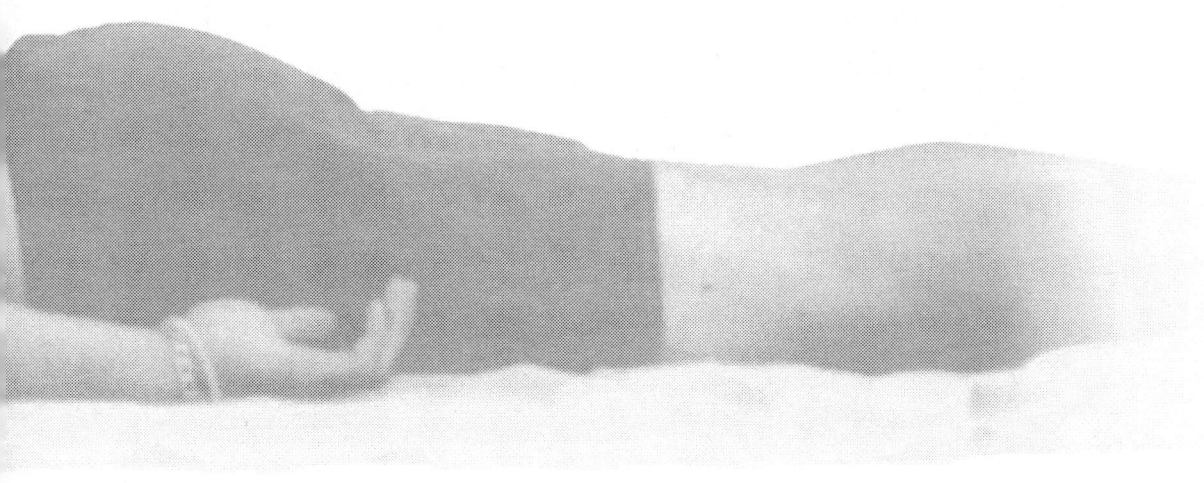

The Twist

The Pose

Sit with the legs out in front of you. Bring the right knee up, placing the right foot flat on the floor. The right arm then comes behind you, palm down to keep your balance and the back up straight.

The left arm lifts up and drops over the right side of the right knee. With an exhalation, lift and turn from the spine, looking behind you to the right.

Hold for a moment, breathe with a soft belly. With an exhalation, come out slowly.

Repeat on the other side.

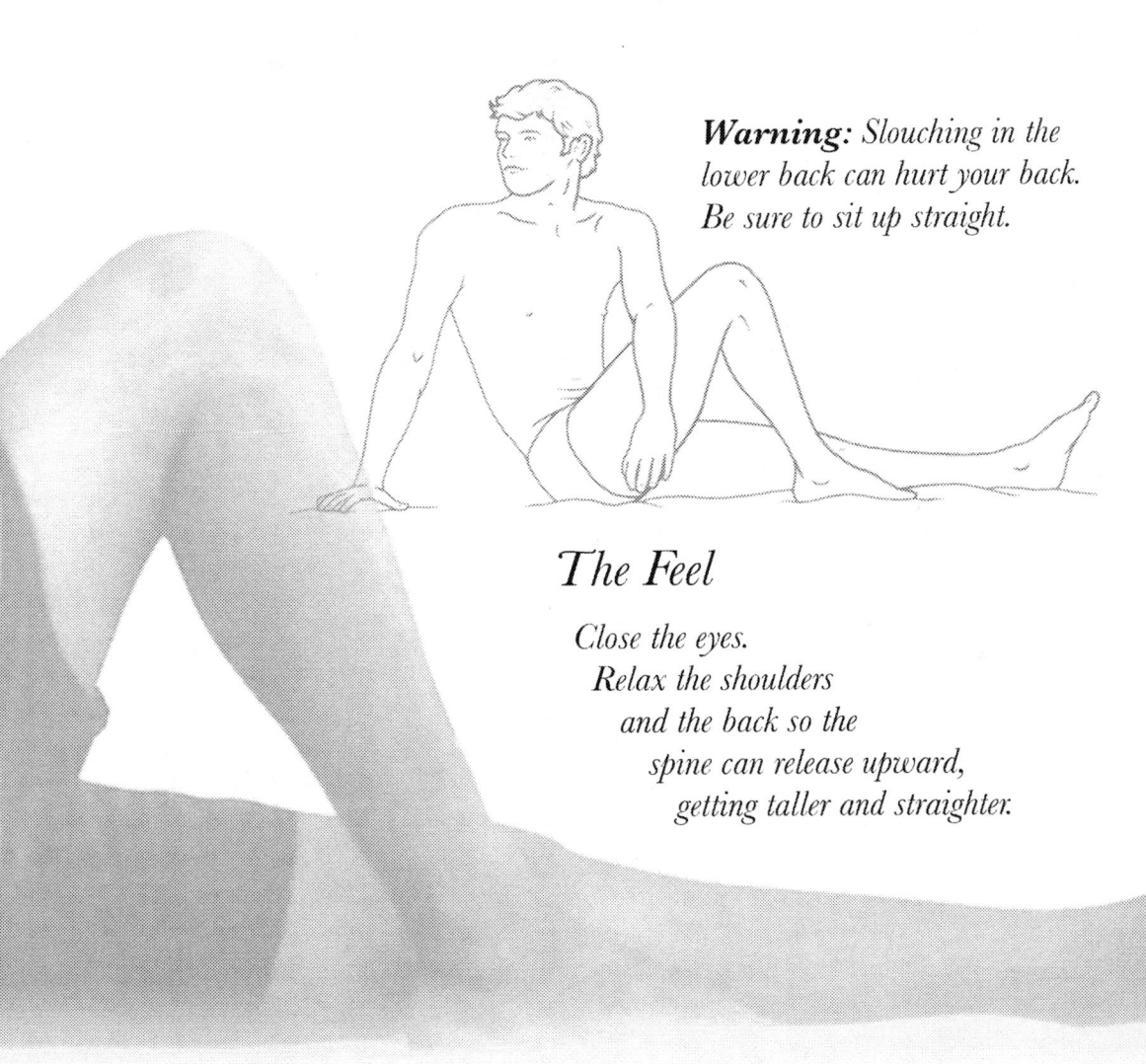

Warning: *Slouching in the lower back can hurt your back. Be sure to sit up straight.*

The Feel

*Close the eyes.
Relax the shoulders
and the back so the
spine can release upward,
getting taller and straighter.*

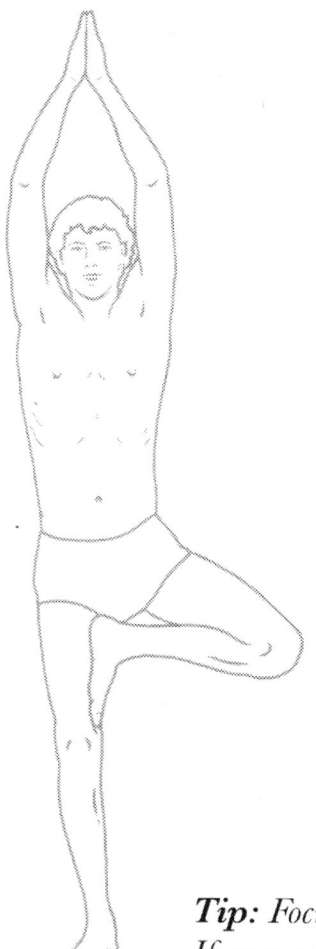

The Tree

The Pose

Come to a standing position.

The secret to balancing poses is a big foot: Point the toes up, place the sole of the foot on the floor, and then drop the ball of the foot and then the toes.

Come forward on the right leg and take a moment to establish your balance.

Place the sole of the left foot on the inside of the right leg - on the ankle, knee or thigh - whatever feels right for you. Then bring the palms up to meet over the head.

Repeat on the other side.

Tip: *Focus the eyes on a single point in front of you. If your mind concentrates, it will help steady the pose.*

The Feel

When balanced, relax the shoulders down and back, so the neck and spine release upwards.

The Dove

The Pose

Kneel and sit back on the legs. Then, sit the buttocks on the floor over to the left, so both feet are to the right. Bring your left arm up (the arm opposite your feet) and hold it by the wrist. Gently lean over towards the right (towards your feet).

Close the eyes. Release the belly.

Hold only as long as feels good.

With an inhalation, come up.

Repeat on other side.......

Tip: *Move slowly into the pose. You will go deeper beginning with a relaxed under-stretch, than rushing into a tight stretch.*

The Feel
Don't hunch forward - the chest is up and proud. Feel the stretch - you needn't rip or tear the muscles.

The Final Relaxation

The Pose

Slowly lie down on the back. Let the feet fall apart so the legs feel relaxed. Legs just far enough apart so the lower back is free of pressure. Lift the shoulders slightly. Put them down slowly. Relax the jaw where it meets the ears. Drop the tongue to the back of the mouth. Let the eyes become soft, unfocused, like in sleep. Relax the abdomen so the breath is free and easy. Let go of all the muscles of the face, the arms and the legs. Let go of the torso, especially the lower back - let it open up. The whole body becomes soft as water. Let the mind sink into the body and come to rest in the feelings, like the rising and falling of the breath.

Relax for 10 to 20 minutes.

Tip: *Cover yourself with a blanket, to keep warm and comfortable. If the Relaxation pose is uncomfortable, you can always do the Reverse Relaxation.*

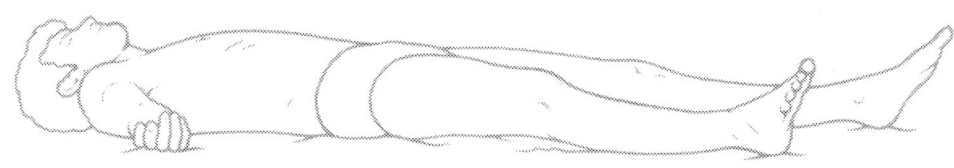

The Feel

Stillness of the body is the key to deep relaxation.
Try not to fidget. The longer the body is still, the deeper the muscles relax and the more the body heals. Imagine floating in a warm bath - that good feeling of warm water all around you, softening the body. Let the mind unfocused, like the moment just before you fall asleep.

No concrete thoughts, no business.

Let thoughts that enter your mind, exit.
Rest in this pleasant, quiet moment -
drifting off into infinite space -
your body filled with a
peaceful, healing
energy.

Last words

*It's easy to lose ourselves and what's really
important to us. Caught in the rush of life,
we lose touch with our sense of purpose and even
well-being. It is important to take time everyday,
to be calm, to be still. Stillness and silence nourish
the soul and let us hear its quiet guidance.*

*You deserve happiness.
By taking the time to take care of yourself,
you have more to offer others.*

Thank you...

Elsie and Evan,
you are the light and warmth that I live for.

Cindy Koelsch,
without your generosity this book would not be here.
It was your kindness and inspiration that saw it through to the end.

Kathy Brownlee and Janis Apted,
my good friends, your selfless advice and help are in these pages.

Eric Mahar,
your friendship and music say it all.

To all my students,
for your years of support and friendship.

To you, my dearest reader,
may you find in life what will make you happiest.

About the Author

Neal Arbic began practicing and studying Yoga over 20 tears ago. Since 1990, he has been a full time Yoga instructor. He has taught thousands of people, including children, seniors, people with disabilities, and the blind. He has been offered positions with corporations such as Husky, Orenda Aerospace and Ford. He turns down many requests so he can look after his young son. He lives with his wife and son, and teaches in Ontario, Canada.

To learn more you can visit:
www.BecomingPeace.NET

A percentage of all the author's profits are donated to the Sri Ram Orphanage in Hardwar, India. The orphanage is dedicated to providing a stable, loving family atmosphere to abandoned or neglected children. The orphanage accepts both infants and older children.

For more information visit:
www.sriramfoundation.org

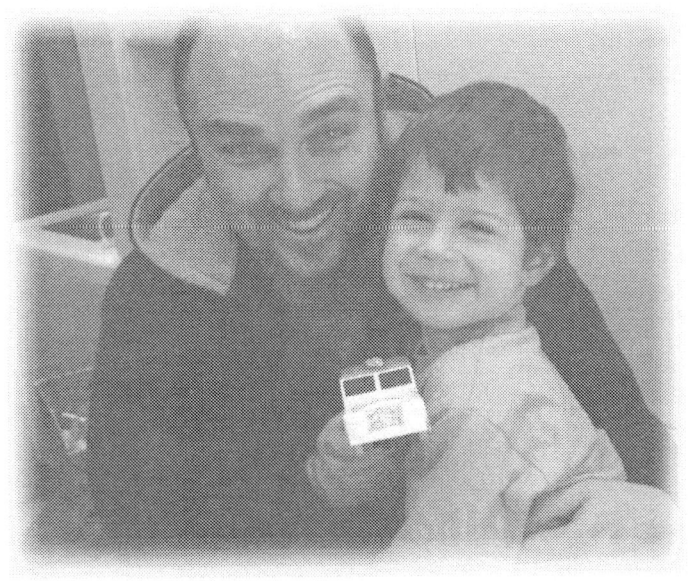

Neal with son Evan

How to use the CD

The Wisdom of Yoga for Everyday Life
To create an intimate space, track 1 is a musical selection from Neal's CD, *Deep Relaxation*. Listen to it while reading the first section, *The Wisdom of Yoga for Everyday Life*.

How to Meditate
Track 2, 3, and 4 are introductions to meditation and track 5 is a ten minute meditation. All tracks are selections from Neal's CD, *Peaceful Meditations*.

A Relaxing Yoga Class
Track 6 is an introduction to the yoga poses and track 7 is a twenty-five minute yoga class with all the poses illustrated in this book. These tracks are selections from Neal's *Relaxing Yoga* CD series.

All music by Eric Mahar.

The complete versions of Neal's CDs are available through

BecomingPeace.Net

ISBN 1412039029